Reproductive Physiology

Fertility and Infertility

Akmal El-Mazny

CONTENTS

INTRODUCTION

The reproductive system consists of the hypothalamic-pituitary unit, the gonads (testes or ovaries), the reproductive tract, and the external genitalia.

The functions of the reproductive system are to produce and deliver gametes (spermatozoa or oocytes) for sexual reproduction, and produce hormones that regulate reproductive function and secondary sex characteristics.

Abnormalities in the physiologic function affect the development and delivery of gametes, and potential fertility.

Male infertility may be due to abnormalities of hormonal control, testicular function, or sperm transport or delivery.

Female infertility can be divided into several categories: ovarian, tubal and peritoneal, uterine, cervical, and other.

This book provides a comprehensive review of the reproductive physiology; emphasizing hormonal control, gamete production, fertilization, implantation, and embryonic development.

By developing a clear understanding of what is normal, you will better understand the abnormalities affecting fertility and the mechanisms behind treatment.

MALE REPRODUCTIVE PHYSIOLOGY

The male reproductive system is a network of external and internal organs that has two major functions:

– Produce and deliver spermatozoa, for sexual reproduction.

– Produce hormones that regulate reproductive function and secondary sex characteristics.

Sperm produced in the testes is transported through the epididymis, ductus deferens, ejaculatory duct, and urethra.

The seminal vesicles, prostate gland, and bulbourethral gland produce seminal fluid that accompany and nourish the sperm as it is emitted from the penis during ejaculation and throughout the fertilization process.

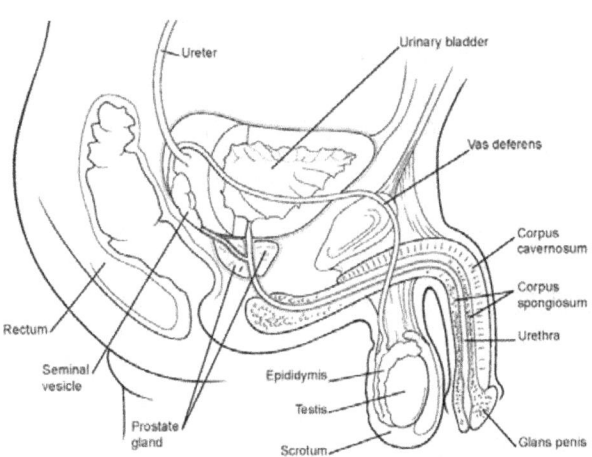

Male Reproductive System

HORMONAL CONTROL

Several hormones control testes function:

− GnRH stimulates the pituitary to synthesize and release LH and FSH.

− LH stimulates Leydig cells to synthesize testosterone.

− FSH maintains Sertoli cell function.

Effects of Testosterone

Testosterone has significant reproductive and nonreproductive effects throughout the male life cycle.

Before birth, testosterone masculinizes the reproductive tract and external genitalia and promotes descent of the testes into the scrotum.

For sex-specific tissues, testosterone promotes growth and maturation of the reproductive system at puberty, is essential for spermatogenesis, and maintains the reproductive tract throughout adulthood.

Other reproductive effects include development of the sex drive at puberty and control of gonadotropin hormone secretion; secondary sex characteristics are also testosterone-dependent.

Testosterone induces the male pattern of hair growth (such as the beard), causes the voice to deepen due to thickening of the vocal cords, and promotes muscle growth responsible for the male body configuration.

Nonreproductive actions of testosterone include a protein anabolic effect, promotion of bone growth at puberty and closure of the epiphyseal plates.

Pituitary Feedback

Testosterone provides negative feedback to the pituitary to decrease LH and FSH levels, and to the hypothalamus to decrease GnRH production.

Inhibin, produced by Sertoli cells, is responsible for the remainder of the inhibition of FSH production.

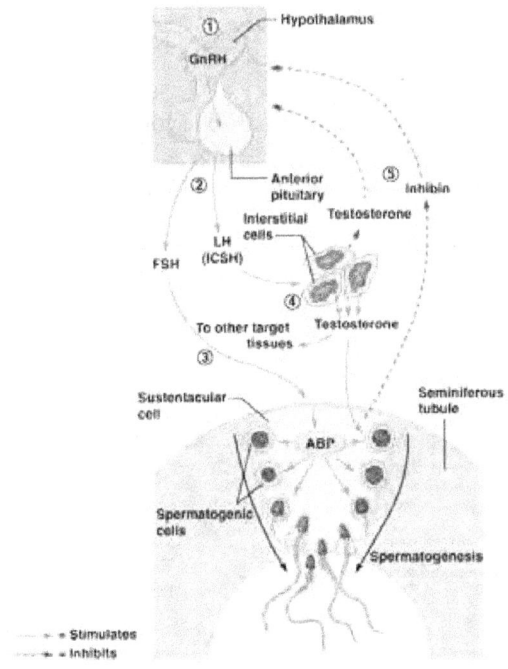

Hormonal Control of Testicular Function

SPERMATOGENESIS

Beginning at puberty, spermatogenesis occurs continuously and repeatedly within folds of the Sertoli cells.

Spermatogonia (the sperm stem cells) lie at the base of the Sertoli cells and proliferate through mitosis to produce daughter cells that enter spermatogenesis.

In the two-step reduction division process of meiosis, spermatocytes and spermatids develop.

Spermatids are haploid, containing only one copy of each chromosome.

As the germ cells divide and mature, they move away from the base of the tubule toward the apical surface of Sertoli cells.

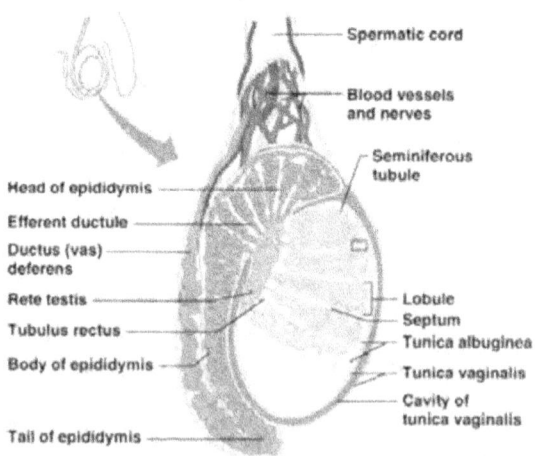

Seminiferous Tubules

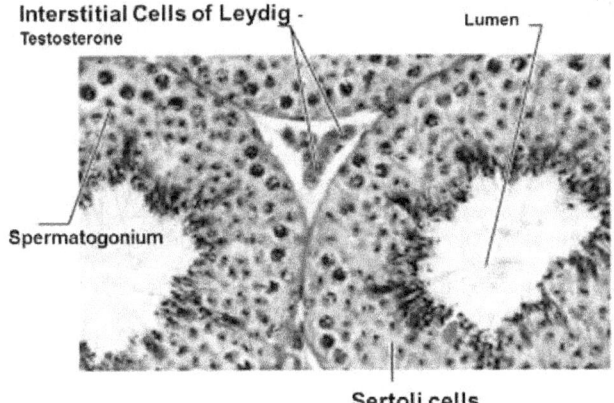

Cell Types within the Testes

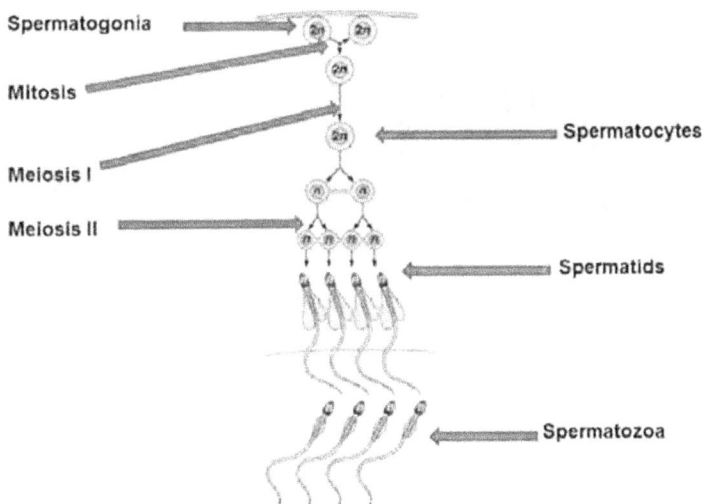

Spermatogenesis

Spermiogenesis

Following meiosis, spermiogenesis is the maturation process in which the round spermatids are transformed into elongated spermatozoa with tails.

The spermatid nucleus condenses and most cytoplasm is lost; the Golgi apparatus moves to one side of the nucleus, forming an acrosome that surrounds the top two thirds of the nucleus (in the head).

Cell microtubules organize into a flagellar apparatus to form the tail for motility, and mitochondria for movement.

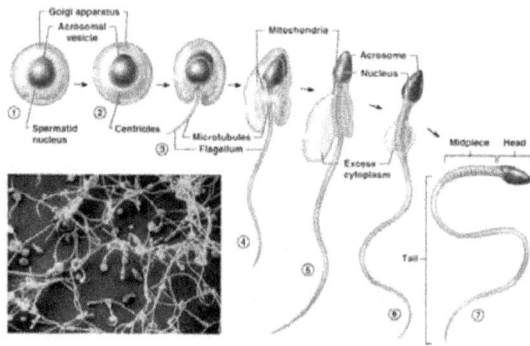

Spermiogenesis

Spermiation

Spermiation is the process in which fully developed but non-motile spermatozoa are released from the Sertoli cells and propelled out of the tubules into the collecting tubules, rete testis and then the epididymis.

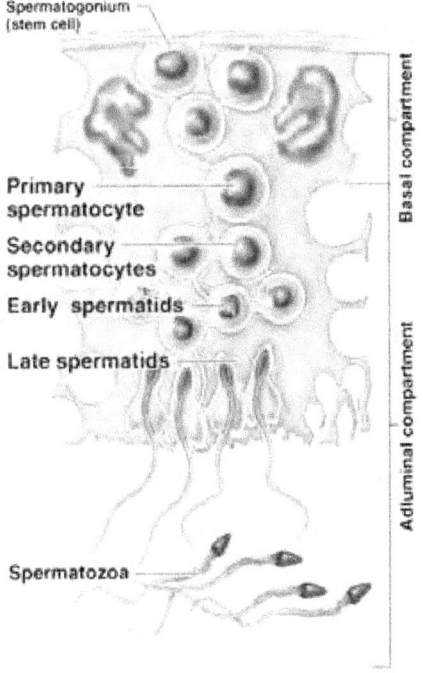

Spermiation

Mature Sperm

Mature sperm have a head, which consists primarily of the nucleus containing genetic information.

The acrosome is a specialized lysosome, containing about 20 different enzymes, which are needed for penetration of the ovum during fertilization.

The acrosome covers the anterior third of the nucleus in a mature sperm.

In the midpiece are mitochondria to provide the energy required for the movement of the tail.

The tail grows out of one of the centrioles; movement results from the sliding of the microtubules.

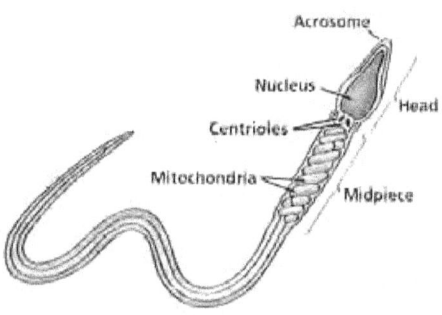

Mature Sperm

Normal Sperm Morphology

Normal sperm morphology is defined by multiple parameters:

– The head is oval shaped, 4-5 microns long, 2-3 microns wide, the length-to-width ratio is 1.5 to 1.75, and a well-defined acrosome makes up 40 to 70% of the head area.

– The midpiece is intact and there is no cytoplasmic droplet.

– The tail is 45 microns long, and is not bent or coiled.

Sperm Abnormalities

Sperm abnormalities are scored in four categories:

− For the head, abnormal characteristics include large, small, tapered, pyriform, amorphous, vacuolated, bicephalic, and acrosome defects.

− In the neck and midpiece, a distended or irregular midpiece, thin midpiece (no mitochondria), and bent or absent tail are abnormal.

− Abnormal tails may be short, multiple, hairpin, broken, or coiled.

− If there is a cytoplasmic droplet attached at the midpiece, the spermatozoon is considered immature.

Manual Assessment of Sperm Motility

Qualitative evaluation of forward motion:

0 = immotile.

1 = tail movement with no forward movement of the sperm.

2 = weak forward progression.

3 = active tail movement with good forward progression.

4 = vigorous tail movement with rapid forward progression.

S<small>PERM</small> T<small>RANSPORT</small>

For each testis there is a duct system; the function of these ducts is testosterone-dependent.

The cells absorb fluid from the testis and remove particulate matter by endocytosis.

The epididymis is where sperm mature, concentrate and are stored for five to six days in this segment of the tract.

The vas deferens is a secondary storage site for spermatozoa; its epithelium has important absorptive and secretory functions.

The other components of the duct system are the ejaculatory duct and the urethra.

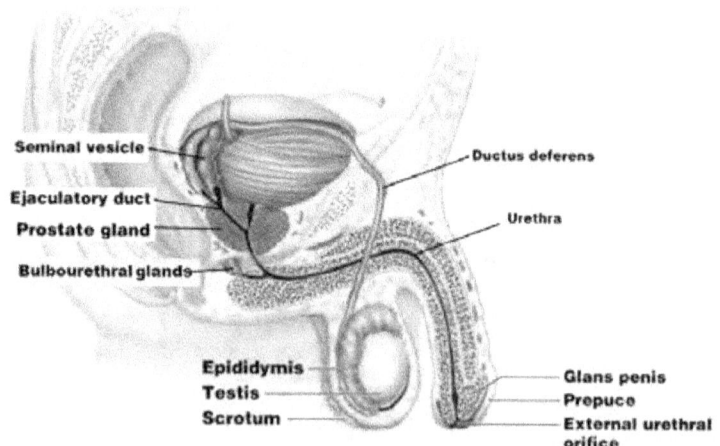

Duct System

Accessory glands include the seminal vesicle, prostate gland and bulbourethral glands.

The seminal vesicle provides precursor proteins responsible for semen coagulation, supplies fructose to nourish the ejaculated sperm and secretes prostaglandins that stimulate motility.

The prostate gland secretes proteolytic enzymes to liquefy coagulum after ejaculation, alkaline fluid to neutralize acidic vaginal secretions and the high zinc content is antimicrobial.

The bulbourethral glands, also known as Cowper's glands, secrete mucus for lubrication.

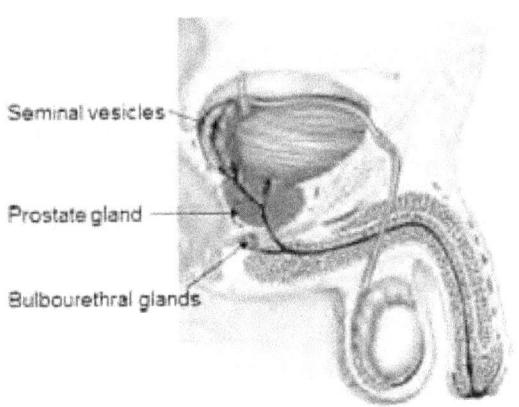

Accessory Glands

ERECTION AND EJACULATION

In the relaxed state, the central arteries in the cavernosa are constricted, limiting blood inflow; blood flows through sinusoids, and out through veins.

In the aroused state, impulses from the brain and local nerves cause the central arteries to dilate and the muscles of the corpora cavernosa to relax.

The blood fills the sinusoids to compress the veins, reducing venous outflow and causing an erection.

As the tunica albuginea expands it compresses exiting veins to help trap blood in the corpora cavernosa, thereby sustaining the erection.

Emission is a sympathetic and parasympathetic (S2-S4) event causing peristaltic waves up the vas deferens and contractions from the seminal vesicles and prostate gland to expel contents to the prostatic urethra.

Ejaculation is expulsion of the semen in the prostatic urethra distally down the urethra.

Ejaculation occurs by expulsion of the contents of the bulbourethral glands, followed by the fluid from the epididymis and prostate, accounting for about 30% of volume and the highest sperm concentration.

Lastly, the seminal vesicles empty and produce the largest portion of the seminal volume.

Semen is an admixture of sperm cells and secretions from the male accessory sex glands that combine at the time of ejaculation.

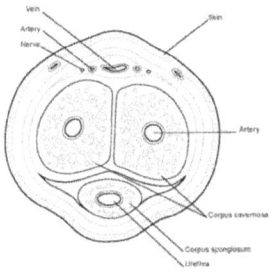

Cross-section of the Penis

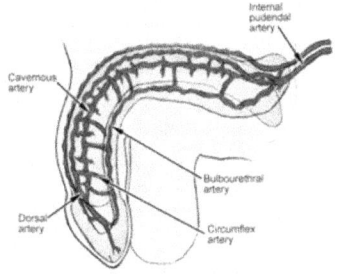

Arterial Supply of the Penis

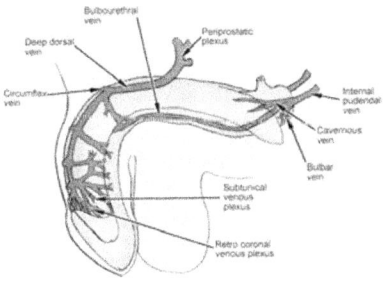

Venous Drainage of the Penis

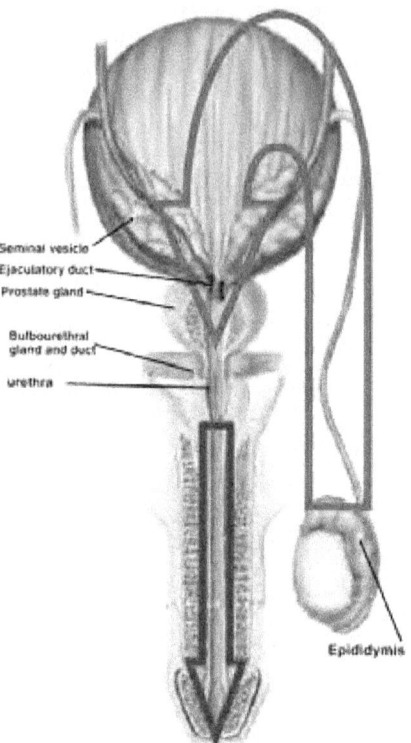

Seminal vesicle
Ejaculatory duct
Prostate gland
Bulbourethral
gland and duct
urethra

Epididymis

Mechanism of Ejaculation

MALE INFERTILITY

Infertility is defined by the World Health Organization (WHO) as the absence of conception after at least 12 months of unprotected intercourse.

An estimated 10-15% of couples meets this criterion and are considered infertile.

Isolated conditions of the female are responsible for infertility in 35% of cases, isolated conditions of the male in 30%, conditions of both the male and female in 20%, and unexplained causes in 15%.

A male factor may be due to hormonal abnormalities resulting in decreased sperm production, abnormalities of testicular function or abnormal sperm transport or delivery.

The initial evaluation of the male patient should be rapid, noninvasive, and cost-effective, as nearly 70% of conditions that cause infertility in men can be diagnosed with history, physical examination, and semen and hormonal analysis alone.

More detailed, invasive, and expensive studies can then be ordered if necessary.

Treatment options are based on the underlying etiology and range from optimizing semen production and transportation with medical therapy or surgical procedures to complex assisted reproduction techniques.

CAUSES

Male infertility may be due to abnormalities of hormonal control, testicular function, or sperm transport or delivery.

Pretesticular Causes

Pretesticular causes of infertility include congenital or acquired diseases of the hypothalamus, pituitary, or peripheral organs that alter the hypothalamic-pituitary axis.

−Kallmann syndrome.

−Prader-Willi syndrome.

−Laurence-Moon-Biedl syndrome.

−Prolactinoma.

−Isolated LH deficiency.

−Isolated FSH deficiency.

−Thalassemia.

−Cushing disease.

Testicular Causes

Primary testicular problems may be chromosomal or nonchromosomal.

While chromosomal failure is usually caused by abnormalities of the sex chromosomes, autosomal disorders are also observed.

Chromosomal Abnormalities

−Klinefelter syndrome (47, XXY).

−XX male.

−XYY male.

−Noonan Syndrome.

−Mixed gonadal dysgenesis (45, X / 46, XY).

−Y-chromosome microdeletions.

−Bilateral anorchia (vanishing testis syndrome).

−Down syndrome.

−Myotonic muscular dystrophy.

−Congenital deficiency of testosterone production.

Nonchromosomal Testicular Failure

−Varicocele.

−Cryptorchidism.

−Androgen insensitivity syndrome (AIS).

−Sertoli-cell-only syndrome.

−Trauma.

−Orchitis.

−Chemotherapy.

−Radiotherapy.

−Idiopathic causes.

Posttesticular Causes

Posttesticular causes of infertility include problems with sperm transportation through the ductal system, either congenital or acquired.

Additionally, the sperm may be unable to cross the cervical mucus or may have ultrastructural abnormalities.

−Congenital blockage of the ductal system.

−Congenital bilateral absence of the vas deferens (CBAVD).

−Acquired ductal obstruction.

−Antisperm antibodies.

−Ejaculatory duct obstruction.

−Ejaculatory disorders.

−Erectile dysfunction.

EVALUATION

The initial step in the evaluation of an infertile male is to obtain a thorough medical history and physical examination.

History

The history should include consideration of the following:

− Duration of infertility.

− Previous fertility in the patient and the partner.

− Timing of puberty (early, normal, or delayed).

− Childhood urologic disorders or surgical procedures.

− Current or recent acute or chronic medical illnesses.

− Sexual history.

− Testicular cancer and its treatment.

− Social history (eg, smoking and alcohol use).

− Medications.

− Family history.

− Respiratory disease.

− Environmental or occupational exposure.

− Spinal cord injury.

Examination

The physical examination should include a thorough inspection of the following:

− Testicles (for bilateral presence, size, consistency, symmetry).

− Epididymis (for presence bilaterally, as well as any induration, cystic changes, enlargement, tenderness).

− Vas deferens (for presence bilaterally, defects, segmental dysplasia, induration, nodularity, swelling).

− Spermatic cord (for varicocele).

− Penis (for anatomic abnormalities, strictures, or plaques).

− Rectum (for abnormalities of the prostate or seminal vesicles).

− Body habitus.

− Depending on the findings from the history, detailed examination of other body functions may also be warranted.

Investigations

The semen analysis is the cornerstone of the male infertility workup and includes assessment of the following:

− Semen volume (normal, 1.5-5 mL).

− Semen quality.

− Sperm density (normal, >15 million sperm/mL).

−Total sperm motility (normal, >40% of sperm having normal movement).

−Sperm morphology (sample lower limit for percentage of normal sperm is 4%).

−Signs of infection: increased number of white blood cells (WBCs) in the semen may be observed in patients with infectious or inflammatory processes.

−Other variables (eg, levels of zinc, citric acid, acid phosphatase, or alpha-glucosidase).

Other laboratory tests that may be helpful include the following:

−Hormonal analysis (FSH, LH, TSH, testosterone, prolactin).

−Antisperm antibody test.

−Genetic testing (karyotype, CFTR, AZF deletions if severe oligospermia (<5 million sperm/mL).

Imaging studies employed in this setting may include the following:

−Scrotal ultrasonography.

−Transrectal ultrasonography.

−Vasography.

Indications for performing a postcoital test include semen hyperviscosity, increased or decreased semen volume with good sperm density, or unexplained infertility.

If the test result is normal, consider sperm function tests, such as the following:

− Capacitation assay.

− Acrosome reaction assay.

− Sperm penetration assay.

− Hypoosmotic swelling test.

− Inhibin B level.

− Vitality stains.

Testicular biopsy is indicated in azoospermic men with a normal-sized testis and normal findings on hormonal studies to evaluate for ductal obstruction and to retrieve sperm.

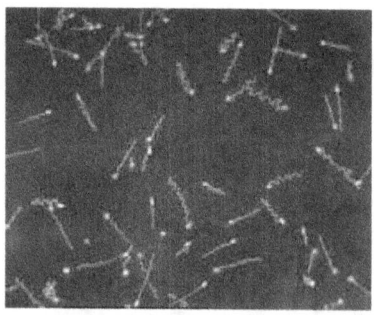

Semen Analysis

TREATMENT

Treatment options are based on the underlying etiology and range from medical therapy or surgical procedures to complex assisted reproduction techniques (ART).

Medical

The following causes of infertility, if identified, can often be treated by medical means:

−Endocrinopathies.

−Poor semen quality or number.

−Infections.

−Antisperm antibodies.

−Retrograde ejaculation.

−Lifestyle issues.

Surgical

Surgical interventions to be considered include the following:

−Varicocelectomy.

−Vasovasostomy or vasoepididymostomy.

−Transurethral resection of the ejaculatory ducts.

−Sperm retrieval techniques (MESA, PESA, TESE).

<u>Assisted Reproduction Techniques (ART)</u>

ART used to treat infertility include the following:

– Intrauterine insemination (IUI).

– In vitro fertilization (IVF).

– Gamete intrafallopian transfer (GIFT).

– Zygote intrafallopian transfer (ZIFT).

– Intracytoplasmic sperm injection (ICSI).

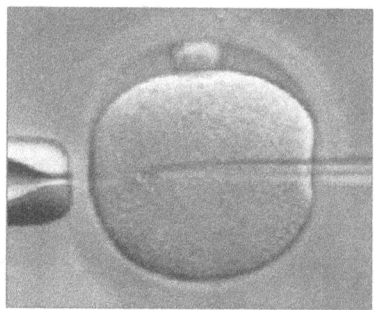

Intracytoplasmic Sperm Injection (ICSI)

FEMALE REPRODUCTIVE PHYSIOLOGY

The female reproductive system is a complicated but fascinating subject.

It has the capability to function intimately with nearly every other body system for the purpose of reproduction.

The female reproductive system consists of the hypothalamic-pituitary unit, the ovaries, the reproductive tract, and the external genitalia.

The functions of the female reproductive system are to produce and deliver oocytes, for sexual reproduction, and produce hormones that regulate reproductive function and secondary sex characteristics.

The female reproductive organs can be subdivided into the internal and external genitalia.

The internal genitalia are those organs that are within the true pelvis: the ovaries, fallopian tubes, uterus, cervix, and vagina.

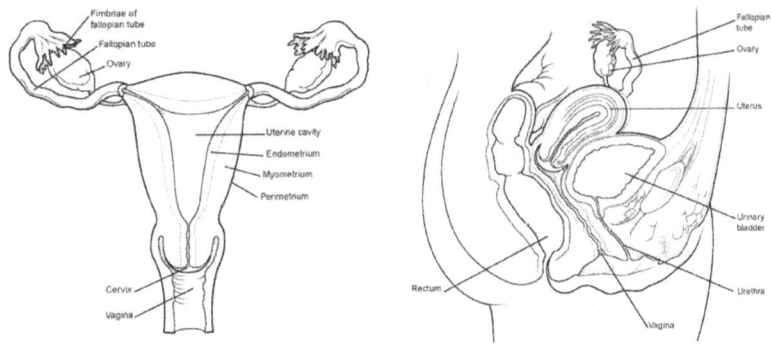

Female Reproductive System

HORMONAL CONTROL

There are four major functional compartments involved in reproduction, each has a specific function: the hypothalamus, the pituitary gland and the ovaries, which compose the hypothalamic-pituitary-ovarian (HPO) axis; and the hormonally-responsive functional endometrium lining the uterus.

In the presence of low levels of estrogen, the arcuate nucleus of the hypothalamus releases gonadotropin-releasing hormone.

This hormone signals the anterior pituitary to produce the gonadotropins LH and FSH.

These gonadotropins in turn induce the development and maturation of ovarian follicles that contain the actual oocytes.

During the growth process, the follicles produce increased amounts of estradiol.

This increase in estrogen production develops the endometrium and thins the increasing amounts of cervical mucus.

When the estradiol level reaches an appropriate level, generally when the follicle is mature, the pituitary releases a large amount of LH.

LH surge causes the final maturation of the oocyte and stimulates the event of ovulation.

After the oocyte is released, that is, ovulation occurs, the sac containing the oocyte undergoes metamorphosis with growth of new blood vessels and becomes a functioning gland called the corpus luteum.

The corpus luteum produces progesterone in large amounts and estrogen in smaller amounts.

Progesterone stabilizes the endometrium and thickens the cervical mucus.

The lifespan of corpus luteum is about 14 days, unless pregnancy occurs.

If the woman does not conceive in a particular cycle, after 14 days, the corpus luteum stops producing progesterone, the endometrium is no longer stable, and menses begin.

The normal menstrual cycle length is 25 to 35 days; this cyclicity is determined by changing sensitivities of the hypothalamic-pituitary unit to estrogens and progestins.

The HPO axis also involves a negative feedback loop in which gonadal secretions produced in response to pituitary gonadotropins inhibit further secretion of gonadotropins.

The HPO axis in the female also involves a positive feedback loop in which ovarian estrogen produced in response to pituitary FSH enhances pituitary secretion of LH and FSH.

Functional Compartment	Location	Hormone or Function
- Hypothalamus	- Arcuate nucleus	- GnRH
- Anterior pituitary	- Gonadotropin	- FSH
		- LH
- Ovary	- Follicle	- Estradiol
	- Corpus luteum	- Progesterone
		- Inhibin
		- Activin
		- Anti-Mullerian hormone
- Uterus	- Endometrium	- Proliferative
		- Secretory
		- Menses

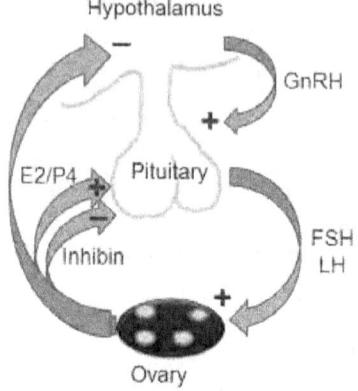

Hypothalamus

GnRH

E2/P4 Pituitary

Inhibin

FSH
LH

Ovary

Hypothalamic-Pituitary-Ovarian (HPO) Axis

Hypothalamus - GnRH

GnRH is synthesized and secreted by neurons in the arcuate nucleus of the hypothalamus and diffuses into the hypothalamic-hypophyseal portal vessels, which transport it to the anterior pituitary gland.

Through pulsatile release, GnRH stimulates the gonadotropes to produce FSH and LH.

The activity of this decapeptide can be modified by changing one or more amino acids; this creates GnRH agonists or antagonists that are often used as adjuncts to infertility and other medical disorders.

Anterior Pituitary - FSH

FSH is a heterodimeric glycoprotein synthesized in gonadotropes in the anterior pituitary.

It has a relatively long half-life in the plasma, normally 3-4 hours; peripheral plasma levels of FSH do not reflect pulsatile GnRH secretion.

FSH stimulates granulosa cells of the ovarian follicle and the luteinized cells of the corpus luteum.

It is considered the critical regulator of follicular development because it is capable of stimulating follicular development by itself.

FSH is suppressed by rising estradiol from the growing follicle; cyclic levels are at their maximum on Day 3 and midcycle surge.

The number of primary follicles which begin to enlarge and respond to FSH is related to the age and total number of oocytes present in the ovary.

Since there is no maturing follicle to suppress FSH, during menopause, FSH is elevated.

Anterior Pituitary - LH

LH is a heterodimeric glycoprotein synthesized in the same gonadotropes in the anterior pituitary as FSH.

LH has a shorter plasma half life (about 20 minutes) than FSH, so peripheral plasma levels do reflect the pronounced pulsatile pattern of GnRH secretion.

LH is secreted in a pulsatile manner:

− In the follicular phase, the pulse interval is normally 90 min.

− In the luteal phase it is about 2 to 3 hours.

LH stimulates mature granulosa cells of the preovulatory follicle and their successor cells, the luteinized cells of the corpus luteum.

LH is capable of maintaining the lifespan of the corpus luteum beyond the normal luteal phase of the menstrual cycle; however, LH is rapidly degraded when administered by injection.

HCG mimics LH, and can therefore stimulate ovulation and support the luteal phase; hCG has a much longer half life and is slower to degrade when administered by injection.

LH has the following stimulatory effects on ovarian cells:

– Increases availability of free cholesterol.

– Stimulates production of androgens in ovarian theca and interstitial cells by increasing enzymes for androgen biosynthesis.

– Increases production of progesterone and estradiol in the corpus luteum.

– Increases plasminogen activator synthesis and secretion in granulosa cells of the preovulatory follicle.

– Stimulates resumption of meiosis in the oocyte at midcycle.

Ovary - Sex Steroids

Although the ovary secretes many substances steroid hormones including androgens, estrogens and progestins, appear to be among the most important.

Androgens are synthesized in the theca and interstitial cells and are important as substrates for estrogen biosynthesis.

The adrenal glands are the principal source of circulating androgens (dehydroepiandrosterone, androstenedione, and testosterone) in women.

The increase in synthesis of adrenal androgens at puberty (called adrenarche) stimulates the development of axillary, pubic and facial hair.

High levels of androgens suppress progesterone synthesis in granulosa cells.

Although the ovaries and adrenals produce similar quantities of androstenedione and testosterone, most of the ovarian androgens are converted to estrogens in the ovaries and in peripheral tissues.

Most of the testosterone in the plasma of the adult female is formed by peripheral conversion of androstenedione by peripheral 17β-hydroxysteroid dehydrogenase.

Estradiol is considered the most important product of the granulosa cells of the developing follicle; estrone is a less active estrogen than estradiol.

Estradiol concentrations in plasma reach a peak during the late follicular phase, decline after ovulation and then rise again during the luteal phase.

Progesterone is considered the most important product of the corpus luteum.

Ovary - Inhibins and Activins

Inhibin is a heterodimeric glycoprotein consisting of an alpha and a beta subunit and is synthesized by granulosa and luteal cells of the ovary.

FSH stimulates granulosa cells to synthesize and secrete inhibin, so that as follicles enlarge, they produce increasing amounts of the hormone.

Inhibin preferentially inhibits synthesis and secretion of FSH but not LH by pituitary gonadotropes (negative feedback).

Inhibin production is low at the beginning of the menstrual cycle, then increases late in the follicular phase and reaches a peak prior to the preovulatory surge of FSH and LH.

After ovulation, inhibin levels decrease slightly, followed by a final rise in the midluteal phase to a level twice that at midcycle.

As the corpus luteum regresses, inhibin levels decline and FSH levels rise with the beginning of the next menstrual cycle.

The ovarian granulosa cells also secrete activin, a dimeric protein consisting of two of the β subunits of inhibin.

Activin amplifies the effect of FSH on granulosa cells in the ovary and also increases the synthesis of the FSH β subunit in the anterior pituitary.

Neuroendocrine Control

– Inhibin, acts on the pituitary to suppress the synthesis and release of FSH, but does not impact LH.

– In the follicular phase, estrogen exerts negative feedback by decreasing the pulse amplitude thereby decreasing FSH and LH pulse amplitude.

– In the luteal phase, progesterone and testosterone decrease GnRH pulse frequency resulting in decreased FSH and LH pulse frequency.

– Testosterone inhibits gonadotropin gene expression in the anterior pituitary; women with elevated serum testosterone levels often do not have normal menstrual cycles.

−GnRH is also inhibited by high concentrations of prolactin; breastfeeding may act as a contraceptive.

−The thyroid can also impact the HPO axis; thyrotropin-releasing hormone (TRH) at high concentrations stimulates the pituitary gland to produce prolactin; patients with hypothyroidism or secondary hyperthyroidism also have decreased gonadotropin secretion.

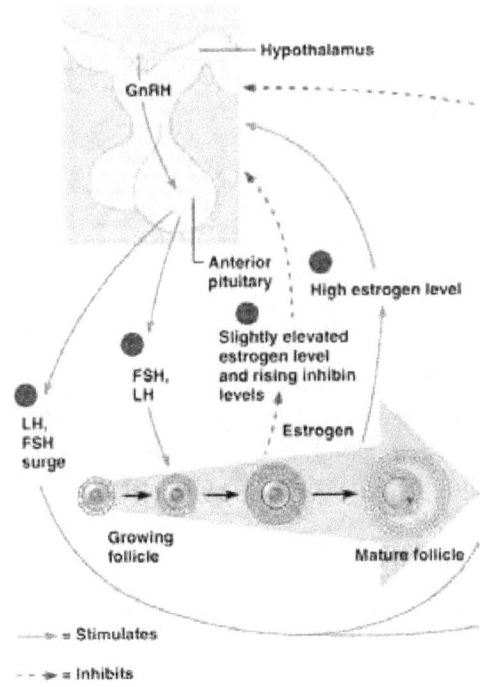

Neuroendocrine Control

OVARIAN CYCLE

The follicle is the basic functional unit of the ovary.

Each follicle consists of an oocyte surrounded by one or more layers of specialized cells (granulosa, theca) which secrete autocrine, paracrine, and endocrine factors.

The follicle grows under the influence of gonadotropins (FSH, LH) and intraovarian regulators (estradiol, IGF-I, activin).

Development from a primordial follicle to a preovulatory follicle takes three to four menstrual cycles.

Follicular Phase

Primordial Follicle

– Primordial follicles are formed during fetal life and are not believed to require gonadotropins for formation; however, females lacking functional FSH receptors have poorly developed ovaries.

– A primordial follicle consists of an oocyte and a single layer of epithelial cells.

– The oocyte is arrested in the first meiotic prophase.

– During the first cycle of development the oocyte grows to about 100 microns in diameter and the epithelial cells enlarge and become cuboidal granulosa cells; at this point, the oocyte is referred to as the "primary follicle".

− FSH receptors are first detectable on the plasma membrane of granulosa cells.

− The granulosa cells respond to FSH by proliferating faster.

Preantral Follicle

− During the first to second cycles of development, the primary follicle progresses to the preantral stage.

− Oocyte meiosis remains arrested.

− The oocyte completes the first step of meiotic maturation, which includes germinal vesicle breakdown and metaphase I after the midcycle LH surge.

− Preantral follicles respond to the midcycle surge of FSH during the second to third cycles of development by growing rapidly; this event is called recruitment.

− All recruited follicles produce sex steroid hormones in amounts proportional to their size and degree of maturation.

− A single follicle, the most mature follicle, becomes dominant.

− The remaining follicles degenerate through a process called atresia.

− The emergence of the single dominant follicle appears to result from the inhibin-induced decline in plasma FSH concentrations.

− Once a dominant follicle is selected, rising serum hormone levels of inhibin and estradiol suppress FSH.

– Local production of estradiol by the dominant follicle amplifies the response to FSH.

– Estradiol synthesis continues to increase exponentially in response to FSH.

Antral Follicle

– Fluid accumulates among the granulosa cells forming the antrum.

– After the antrum is formed, the follicle is termed a "secondary follicle".

Preovulatory Follicle

– During the last cycle of development (third or fourth cycle), the dominant follicle attains its maximal size and the theca layer vascularizes; this represents the "Graafian follicle".

– The oocyte (meiosis still arrested) has the capacity to proceed to metaphase II and complete meiotic maturation after fertilization.

– Granulosa cells of immature follicles have few LH receptors so they don't respond to LH at physiological LH concentrations.

– The theca cells do have LH receptors and they respond to LH.

– One of the actions of FSH on granulosa cells during the follicular phase is to induce LH receptors so that granulosa cells of the preovulatory Graafian follicle become responsive to LH as well as to FSH.

– After the LH/FSH surge prior to ovulation, the granulosa cells initially decrease their LH and FSH receptors and then increase them as the granulosa cells luteinize to become the corpus luteum.

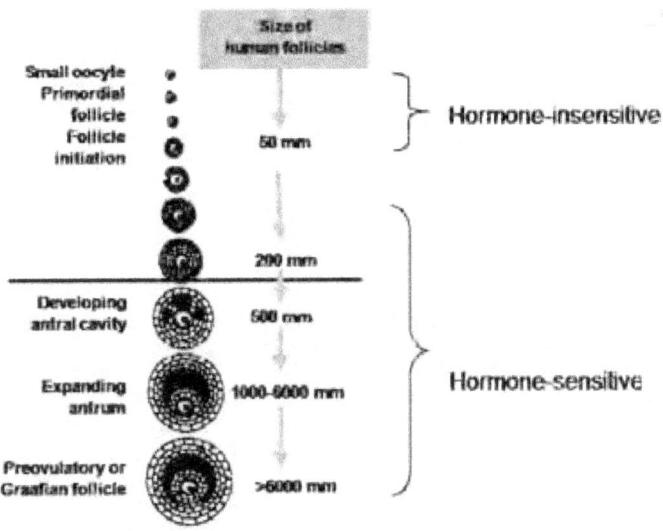

Follicle Development

Ovulation Phase

– LH triggers several processes that culminate in ovulation.

– LH causes a resumption of oocyte meiosis, and metaphase I is completed.

– The first polar body is extruded, and meiosis then halts in metaphase II.

– An increase in follicular pressure, combined with LH-activated breakdown of the follicular wall results in follicular rupture.

– The cumulus-oocyte complex is ovulated 34-36 hours after the onset of the LH surge, and the remaining granulosa and theca cells luteinize.

Luteal Phase

– After ovulation the follicular cells luteinize and form the corpus luteum (literally, yellow body).

– They acquire the capacity to secrete progesterone, and lipid droplets accumulate in the cells.

– If the oocyte is fertilized and implants in the endometrium, the corpus luteum remains active and secretes progesterone in large amounts and estradiol in smaller amounts.

– Progesterone from the corpus luteum prepares the endometrium for implantation and maintains the fetal-placental unit during the first half of the first trimester of pregnancy.

– The corpus luteum requires low levels of LH for continued function.

– LH stimulates the production of progesterone and estradiol, and FSH stimulates the production of estradiol only.

– If fertilization and implantation do not occur, the corpus luteum degenerates (called luteolysis), and progesterone declines within 10 days after ovulation.

– Unlike the variable length of the follicular phase of the menstrual cycle, the luteal phase has a lifespan of about 14 days; this lifespan is due to the fairly consistent lifespan of the corpus luteum.

– However, if pregnancy occurs, the corpus luteum is rescued by hCG that is produced by the implanted trophoblasts.

−LH and hCG are similar in structure; hCG may be thought of as long acting LH.

−In clinical situations hCG injections are used to act like LH, particularly to induce ovulation or stimulate luteal progesterone production.

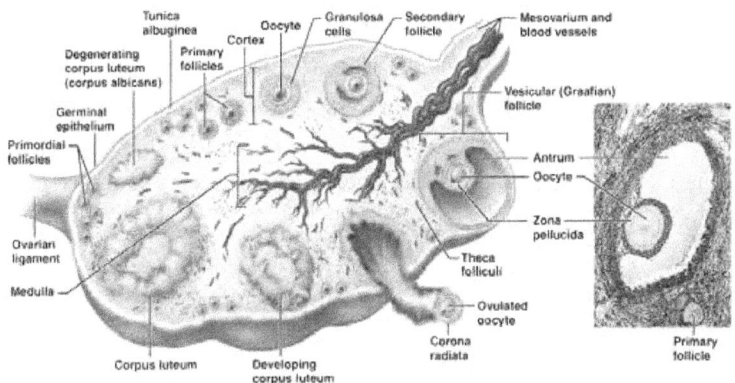

Ovarian Cycle

OOCYTE DEVELOPMENT

The ovaries and germ cells (which develop into oocytes) form during the first few weeks of embryonic life.

These germ cells rapidly divide by a process called mitosis, in which each new daughter cell contains the same number of chromosomes as the parent cell.

During the first trimester of embryonic growth, these preoocyte cells are called oogonium (plural: oogonia).

During the second trimester of life, the 46 chromosomes start to replicate through the process of meiosis but remain within the cell.

At this stage of meiosis, the cell is called a primary oocyte (primitive ovum not yet fully developed).

At this point, further chromosome separation and oocyte development are arrested until after puberty.

These primary oocytes are surrounded by a layer of epithelium that gives rise to the primordial follicles.

About 1700 germ cells are present before migration to the genital ridge begins.

However, these multiply during the process of migration, reaching a peak of 7 million oocytes at midgestation.

The primordial germ cells increase in size early in their development and become oogonia.

At midgestation, they begin the first meiotic division, becoming primary oocytes.

This prophase lasts until just before ovulation, which may occur 12 to 40 or more years later.

In this state, they are no longer capable of multiplication and, in fact, steadily decline in number.

About 400 ova are released through the process of ovulation during a woman's lifetime.

The remaining ova undergo atresia (a normal process affecting the primordial ovarian follicles in which death of the ovum results in degeneration) so that, by the time of the menopause, few are present.

The oocyte remains in this stage until it is either eliminated by atresia or succeeds in reaching the maturation stage and resumption of meiosis (reduction division) at the time of ovulation.

Meiosis has two purposes: reduction to the haploid number of chromosomes to one half of the normal, or 23, and recombination of genetic information.

The first meiotic division, which begins during fetal life, is completed prior to ovulation and produces a secondary oocyte containing 23 chromosomes and the first polar body containing 23 chromosomes, each with 2 daughter chromatids.

A polar body is composed of cell division products that result from meiosis.

The second meiotic division, which is initiated after ovulation, is completed at sperm penetration and produces a mature oocyte containing 23 chromosomes and a polar body containing 23 chromosomes, each with a single chromatid.

When the oocyte and sperm combine at fertilization, the full complement of 46 chromosomes is restored and a new life is created.

The second polar body will degenerate like the first.

As a result of the combined meiotic processes, a single mature oocyte is produced and 2 or 3 polar bodies degenerate.

This is in contrast to the meiotic process in males where a single precursor cell gives rise to 4 mature sperm.

Oocyte Maturation and Ovulation

– Resumption of meiosis begins within the ovarian follicle in response to the LH surge.

– The granulosa cells, that is, the cumulus oophorus, expands.

– The first polar body is extruded and the oocyte progresses into metaphase of the second meiotic division.

– Meiosis stops in metaphase II until fertilization.

Fertilization

Contractions of the oviductal muscles direct the oocyte into the ampulla of the fallopian tube where it remains for about 3 days while the ampullary-isthmic sphincter remains contracted.

The oocytes remain fertile for only 15-18 hours after ovulation while sperm are motile for 24 hours to several days after ejaculation.

When a sperm encounters the zona pellucida, it undergoes an acrosome reaction; this breaks down the acrosomal membrane.

The sperm head membrane binds to the sperm receptor, which is followed by fusion with the oolemma.

Microvilli on the oocyte surface surround the sperm head and the oocyte undergoes the cortical reaction (release of cortical granules).

The zona pellucida hardens and no other sperm can penetrate the oolemma.

The oocyte nucleus completes maturation to yield the female pronucleus and the second polar body; the sperm nucleus forms the male pronucleus.

The corona radiata is the layer of granulosa cells surrounding the oocyte; the zona pellucida is an extracellular layer of proteins surrounding the oocyte.

Egg Activation

Egg activation occurs after fertilization, and involves the completion of the second meiotic division and initiation of embryonic development.

Mitosis begins and there are changes in maternal messenger ribonucleic acids and protein synthesis.

Exocytosis of cortical granules blocks polyspermy and cytoskeletal rearrangement occurs.

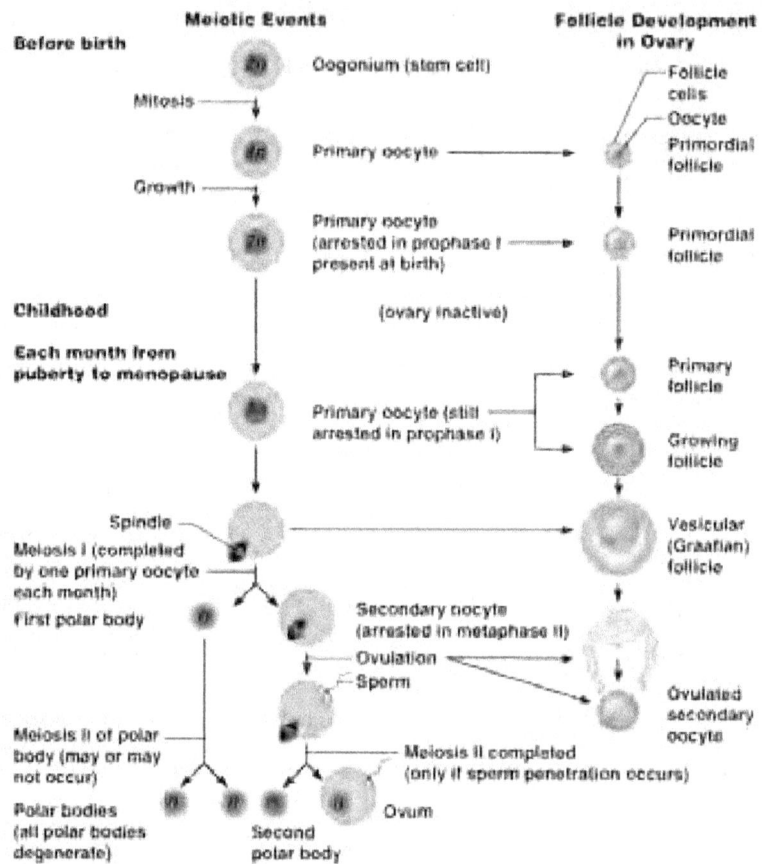

Oocyte Development

FERTILIZATION

The fallopian tubes, or oviducts, function as conduits for the oocyte and spermatozoa, and they provide nutrients for the gametes and early embryo, as well as serving as the site of fertilization.

Ciliated cells at the open, fimbriated end (ostium) direct the oocyte into the infundibulum and down through the ampulla.

Fertilization usually occurs in the distal third of the fallopian tube adjacent to ovary (ampulla).

The zygote is kept in the fallopian tube for about three days by the spastic contractions of the estrogen-dominated isthmus; as progesterone increases, muscle tone decreases.

Oviductal fluid is enriched in lactic acid and bicarbonate, which are important for cleavage of fertilized eggs or zygotes.

Once the zygote divides it is called an embryo; while still in the fallopian tube, the embryo undergoes cleavage division (1-cell to 8-cell), compaction and blastocyst formation before it reaches the uterus.

The inner cell mass of the embryo becomes the fetus and the outer cells become the placenta and fetal membranes.

Peristalsis moves the fertilized oocyte through the tubal isthmus and into the uterus for implantation.

Approximately seven days after fertilization, the blastocyst bursts from the zona pellucida (hatching) and implants in the wall of the uterus.

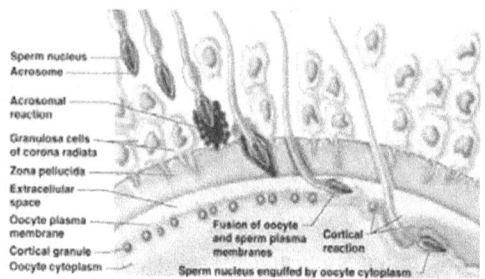

Fertilization

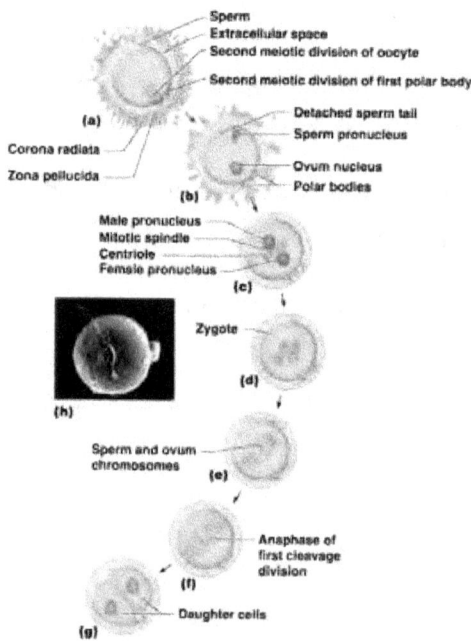

Embryo Cleavage

ENDOMETRIAL CYCLE

Proliferative Phase

The preovulatory follicular phase begins with menses; FSH and LH are released with each GnRH pulse.

Inhibin secretion is low so that FSH, which began to rise late in the luteal phase of the prior cycle, continues to rise.

At the same time, LH levels start to rise slowly.

Several secondary follicles of different sizes are recruited, and they secrete increasing amounts of estrogen and inhibin.

Estrogen and IGF-I increase the sensitivity of the follicle to FSH, while inhibin blunts the pituitary FSH response to GnRH leading to a decrease in plasma FSH.

The follicle most sensitive to FSH continues to develop and becomes the dominant follicle.

Less developed, that is, less sensitive, follicles undergo degeneration (atresia) because of insufficient FSH.

Estrogen decreases the amplitude of GnRH pulses, as well as increases pituitary sensitivity to GnRH.

Estrogen causes proliferation and vascularization of the endometrium, and increases myometrial contractility.

Estrogen also causes the cervical mucus to become clear and thin.

Secretory Phase

When plasma estradiol exceeds 150-200 pg/mL for 36 hours, GnRH triggers a large surge of LH and a small surge of FSH.

The FSH surge recruits new follicles for the next cycle; the LH surge triggers ovulation and luteinization of follicular cells.

The corpus luteum then synthesizes increasing amounts of progesterone, estradiol, and inhibin.

FSH and LH are low, but they maintain the corpus luteum.

Progesterone decreases the frequency of GnRH pulses resulting in a decrease in the frequency of LH pulses.

The LH pulse amplitude increases, however, so that plasma LH remains unchanged.

The post-ovulatory rise in progesterone appears to be responsible for the rise in basal body temperature.

Progesterone decreases myometrial excitability and increases endometrial secretory activity.

The luteal phase has a more constant length than the follicular phase.

Menstrual Phase

If implantation of the blastocyst occurs, the lifespan of the corpus luteum is prolonged by hCG, which is produced by the developing embryo.

If implantation does not occur, the corpus luteum regresses.

Luteal regression begins 14-15 days after ovulation, and progesterone levels decrease to follicular phase levels.

The endometrial lining undergoes ischemic necrosis followed by menses, which is desquamation and bleeding.

Menstruation lasts 3-5 days, and on average, 35 ml of blood + 35 ml serous fluid are lost.

One day before menstruation, when the inhibin levels are low, FSH begins to rise - the proliferative phase is again initiated.

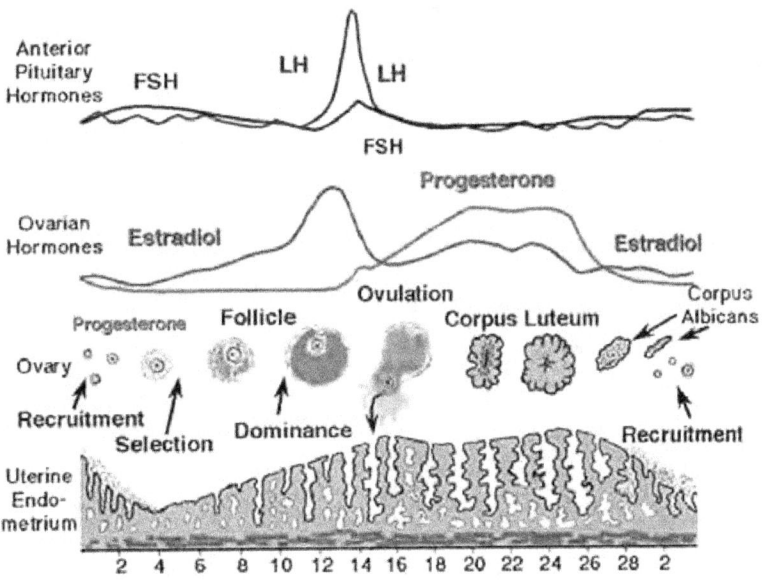

Endometrial Cycle

IMPLANTATION

Approximately seven days after fertilization, the blastocyst bursts from the zona pellucida (hatching) and implants in the wall of the uterus.

Implantation requires prior conditioning of the endometrium by progesterone, which causes the stromal cells to swell and accumulate glycogen, lipids and protein.

The presence of hCG from the blastocyst stimulates the corpus luteum of the maternal ovary to secrete progesterone.

The blastocyst attaches to the uterine fundus at the embryonic pole.

Trophoblast cells then invade through the endometrial epithelium into the endometrial stroma aided by proteases.

Stromal cells decidualize; a process by which they enlarge and become transcriptionally active, and surround the blastocyst.

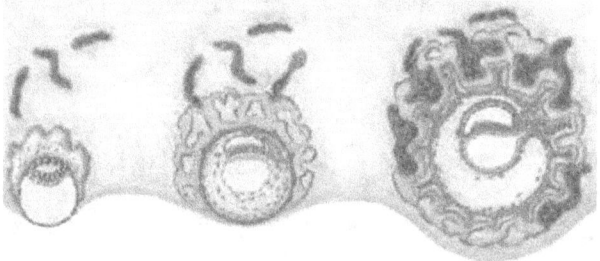

Implantation

EMBRYO DEVELOPMENT

The zygote is kept in the fallopian tube for about three days by the spastic contractions of the estrogen-dominated isthmus; as progesterone increases, muscle tone decreases.

In the fallopian tube, the zygote undergoes cleavage division (1-cell to 8-cell), compaction and blastocyst formation.

The inner cell mass becomes the fetus and the outer cells become the placenta and fetal membranes.

Peristalsis moves the fertilized oocyte through the tubal isthmus and into the uterus for implantation.

Approximately seven days after fertilization, the blastocyst bursts from the zona pellucida, which is called hatching, and implants in the wall of the uterus, which is called nidation.

Implantation requires prior conditioning of the endometrium by progesterone, which causes the stromal cells to swell and accumulate glycogen, lipids and protein.

The presence of hCG from the blastocyst stimulates the corpus luteum of the maternal ovary to secrete progesterone.

The blastocyst attaches to the wall of the uterine fundus at the embryonic pole.

Trophoblast cells then invade through the endometrial epithelium into the endometrial stroma aided by proteases.

Stromal cells decidualize; a process by which they enlarge and become transcriptionally active, and surround the blastocyst.

Within 11 days of fertilization, the trophoblast forms two layers, the cytotrophoblast and the syncytiotrophoblast, containing lacunae.

The placenta forms a barrier to permit exchange of nutrients, gases and wastes with only slight mixing of fetal blood with maternal blood.

Fetal blood cells can normally be found in the maternal circulation in all cases.

As the lacunae enlarge, the trophoblast forms villi, which consist of a vascularized core of cytotrophoblast covered by syncytiotrophoblast.

The trophoblast erodes the maternal spiral arteries, which then flow directly into the intervillous spaces.

The fully developed placenta consists of the following three layers of membranes:

– Amnion (inner), which is a single layer of ectodermal epithelium completely enclosing the embryo;

– Chorion (outer), which surrounds the amniotic sac and includes the villi and trophoblast; and

– The decidua of the maternal endometrium.

The uterofetoplacental circulation is established by about 6 gestational weeks and is completed by 10 weeks, connecting the maternal decidua through the chorionic villi to the fetus via the umbilical vessels.

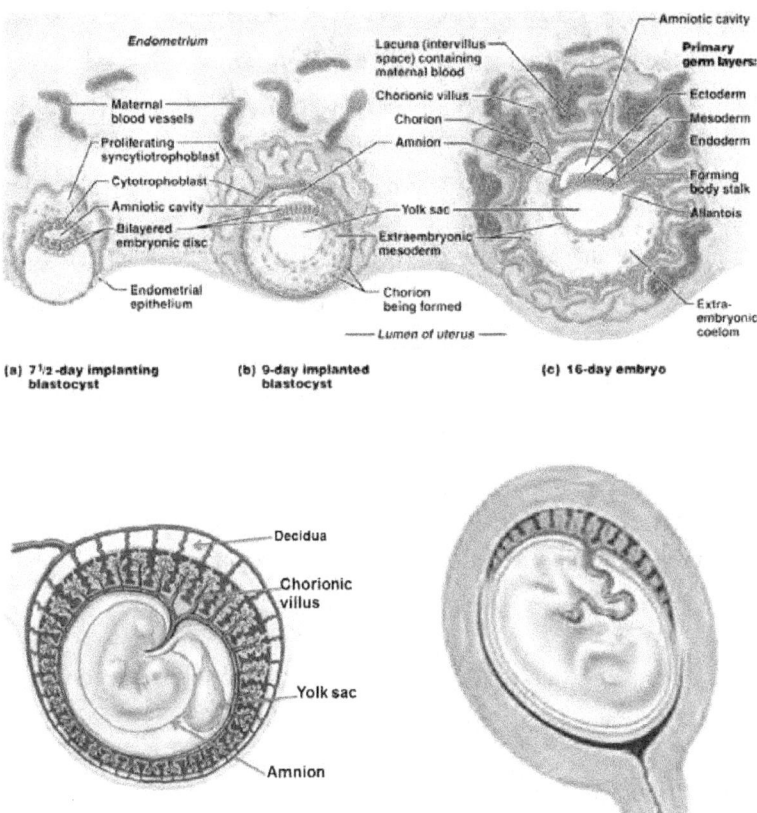

(a) 7¹/₂-day implanting blastocyst

(b) 9-day implanted blastocyst

(c) 16-day embryo

Labels:

Endometrium

Maternal blood vessels

Proliferating syncytiotrophoblast

Cytotrophoblast

Amniotic cavity

Bilayered embryonic disc

Endometrial epithelium

Lacuna (intervillus space) containing maternal blood

Chorionic villus

Chorion

Amnion

Yolk sac

Extraembryonic mesoderm

Chorion being formed

Lumen of uterus

Amniotic cavity

Primary germ layers:

Ectoderm

Mesoderm

Endoderm

Forming body stalk

Allantois

Extra-embryonic coelom

Decidua

Chorionic villus

Yolk sac

Amnion

Embryo Development

FEMALE INFERTILITY

Isolated conditions of the female are responsible for infertility in 35% of cases, isolated conditions of the male in 30%, conditions of both the male and female in 20%, and unexplained causes in 15%.

To understand the rationale for deciding what should be included in a female fertility evaluation, it is helpful to consider what is required in order to establish a normal pregnancy:

– The production of adequate spermatozoa.

– The release of a normal preovulatory oocyte.

– The normal transport of the gametes to the ampullary portion of the fallopian tube (where fertilization occurs).

– The subsequent transport of the cleaving embryo into the endometrial cavity for implantation and development.

Female factor infertility can be divided into several categories: ovarian, tubal and peritoneal, uterine, cervical, and other.

A basic evaluation for female infertility includes an assessment for ovulation, tubal patency, and normality of the uterine cavity.

Management of female factors affecting fertility may include medical treatment, surgical intervention, or assisted reproductive techniques.

CAUSES

Female factors that affect fertility include the following categories:

Ovarian Factors

Alteration in the frequency and duration of the menstrual cycle.

Failure to ovulate is the most common infertility problem

– Polycystic ovarian syndrome (PCOS).

– Hypergonadotropic hypogonadism.

– Hypogonadotropic hypogonadism.

– Prolactin disorders.

– Chromosomal abnormalities.

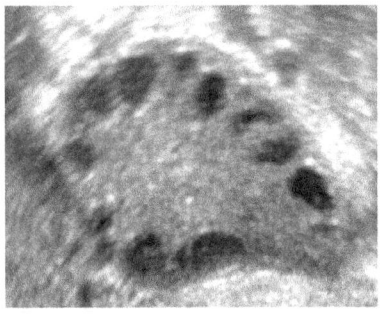 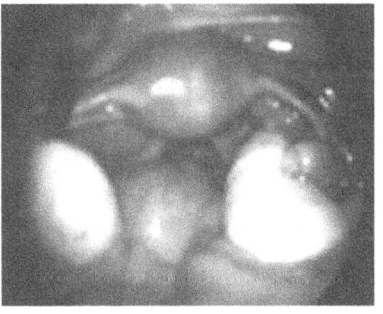

Ultrasonography **Laparoscopy**

Polycystic Ovarian Syndrome (PCOS)

Tubal Factors

Abnormalities or damage to the fallopian tube interferes with fertility and is responsible for abnormal implantation (eg, ectopic pregnancy).

Obstruction of the distal end of the fallopian tubes results in accumulation of the normally secreted tubal fluid, creating distention of the tube with subsequent damage of the epithelial cilia (hydrosalpinx).

Other tubal factors associated with infertility are either congenital or acquired.

Congenital absence of the fallopian tubes can be due to spontaneous torsion in utero followed by necrosis and reabsorption.

Elective tubal ligation and salpingectomy are acquired causes.

Anatomical defects or physiologic dysfunctions of the peritoneal cavity, including infection, adhesions, and adnexal masses, may cause infertility.

Pelvic inflammatory disease (PID), peritoneal adhesions secondary to previous pelvic surgery, endometriosis, and ovarian cyst rupture all compromise the motility of the fallopian tubes or produce blockage of the fimbriae with development of hydrosalpinx.

Large myomas, pelvic masses, or blockage of the cul-de-sac interferes with the accumulation of peritoneal fluid and interferes with the normal oocyte pickup mechanism.

Peri-ovarian adhesions that encapsulate the ovary interfere with the normal oocyte release at ovulation, becoming a mechanical factor for infertility.

Uterine Factors

Uterine factors can be congenital or acquired.

The full spectrum of congenital/müllerian abnormalities varies from total absence of the uterus and vagina (Rokitansky-Küster-Hauser syndrome) to minor defects such as arcuate uterus and vaginal septa (transverse or longitudinal).

The relationship between müllerian anomalies and infertility is not entirely clear except when absolute absence of the uterus, cervix, vagina, or a combination of these occurs.

Premature delivery has been associated with cervical incompetence, unicornuate uterus associated with a blind horn, and septate uterus.

Septate uterus may also be responsible for implantation problems and first-trimester miscarriages.

Endometritis associated with a traumatic delivery, dilatation and curettage, intrauterine device, or any instrumentation (eg, myomectomy, hysteroscopy) of the endometrial cavity may create intrauterine adhesions, with partial or total obliteration of the endometrial cavity.

Intrauterine and submucosal fibroids may be implicated in implantation failure, early miscarriages, premature delivery, and abruptio placentae.

EVALUATION

A complete infertility evaluation is performed according to the woman's menstrual cycle and may take up to 2 menstrual cycles before the etiology is determined.

History

Obtain the following medical history and information:

– Type of infertility (primary or secondary) and its duration.

– History of previous pregnancies and their outcomes; pregnancy intervals; and detailed information about pregnancy loss, pregnancy duration, human chorionic gonadotropin (hCG) level, ultrasonographic data, and presence/absence of fetal heartbeat.

– History of previous infertility evaluation/treatment, including details about frequency of intercourse, use of lubricants (eg, K-Y gel) that could be spermicidal, use of vaginal douches after intercourse, and presence of any sexual dysfunction.

– Menstrual history, frequency, and patterns since menarche, as well as history of weight changes, hirsutism, frontal balding, and acne.

– Male medical history, including previous semen analysis results, history of impotence, premature ejaculation, change in libido, history of testicular trauma, previous relationships, history of any previous pregnancy in female partners, and the existence of offspring from previous female partners.

−Couple's history of sexually transmitted diseases (STDs); surgical contraception (eg, vasectomy, tubal ligation); lifestyle; consumption of alcohol, tobacco, and recreational drugs (amount and frequency); occupation; and physical activities.

−Couple's current medical treatment (if any), reason, and any history of allergies.

−Complete review of systems to identify any endocrinologic or immunologic issue that may be associated with infertility.

Examination

Examination for infertility should include the following:

−Routine records of blood pressure, pulse rate, and temperature (if applicable).

−Height/weight findings to calculate body mass index.

−Head and neck assessment: the presence of exophthalmos can be associated with hyperthyroidism; the presence of epicanthus, lower implantation of ears and hairline, and webbed neck can be associated with chromosomal abnormalities; thyroid gland enlargement/nodules, which may indicate thyroid dysfunction.

−Breast evaluation: Assess breast development and seek any abnormal masses or secretions, especially galactorrhea.

−Abdominal evaluation: Assess for presence of abnormal masses at hypogastrium level.

- Thorough gynecologic evaluation: Assess for hair distribution, clitoris size, Bartholin glands, labia majora/minora, and any condylomata acuminatum or other lesions that could indicate the existence of venereal disease.

- Speculum examination: Obtain a Papanicolaou test and cultures for gonorrhea, chlamydia, Ureaplasma urealyticum, Mycoplasma hominis; assess for cervical stenosis.

- Bimanual examination: Establish direction of the cervix plus size/position of the uterus to exclude the presence of uterine fibroids, adnexal masses, tenderness, or pelvic nodules indicative of infection or endometriosis; assess for defects (eg, absence of vagina and uterus, vaginal septum).

- Extremities evaluation: Exclude malformation (eg, shortness of fourth finger, cubitus valgus), which can indicate chromosomal abnormalities and other congenital defects.

- Dermatologic evaluation: acne, hypertrichosis, and hirsutism.

Investigations

Laboratory, radiologic, and/or surgical assessment of the female includes:

Ovarian Factors

Progesterone levels and ultrasonography to assess ovulation; LH/FSH ratio to assess PCOS; FSH and estradiol levels (or antral follicle count, ovarian volume, and AMH) to assess ovarian reserve; clomiphene citrate challenge test for dynamic ovarian reserve testing.

Tubal Factors

Hysterosalpingogram (HSG) and laparoscopy.

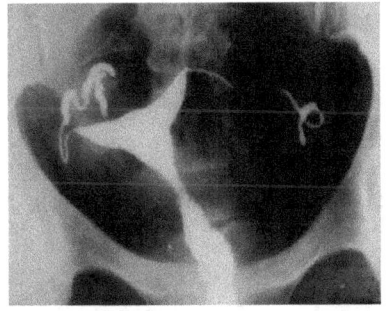
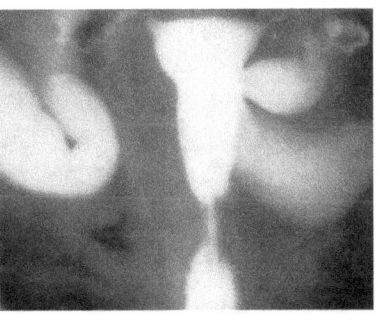

Normal   **Hydrosalpinx**

Hysterosalpingogram (HSG)

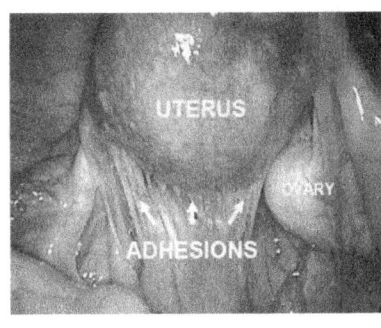
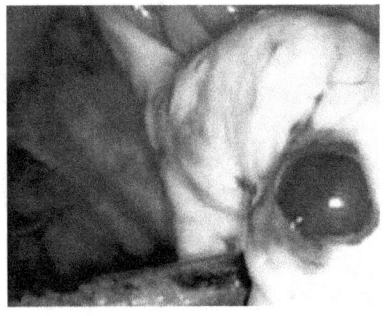

Pelvic Adhesions   **Ovarian Endometriosis**

Laparoscopy

<u>Uterine Factors</u>

Hysterosalpingogram (HSG) - most frequently used to assess endometrial cavity; pelvic ultrasonogram; saline infusion sonogram (SIS); pelvic magnetic resonance imaging; hysteroscopy; and endometrial biopsy.

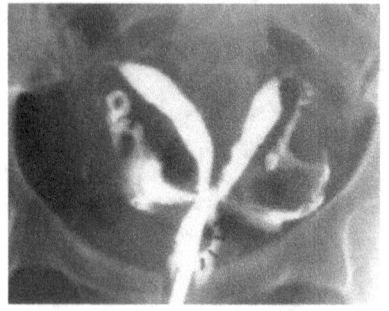 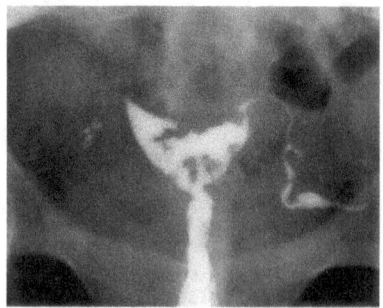

Septate Uterus   **Endometrial Polyps**

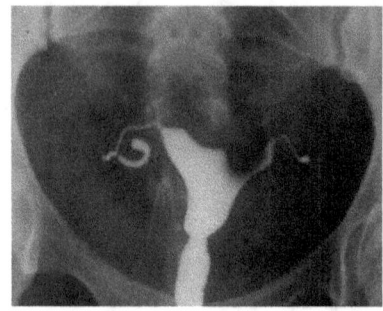 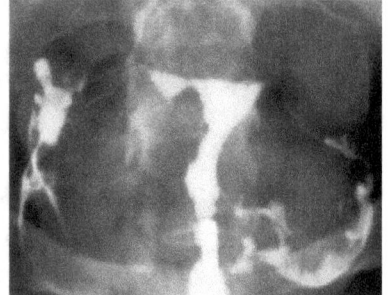

Submucous Fibroid   **Intrauterine Adhesions**

Hysterosalpingogram (HSG)

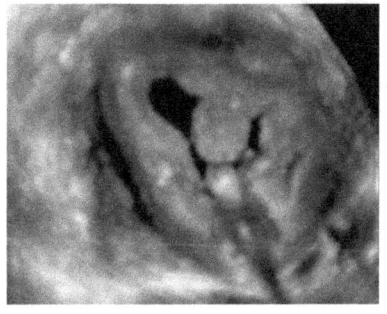
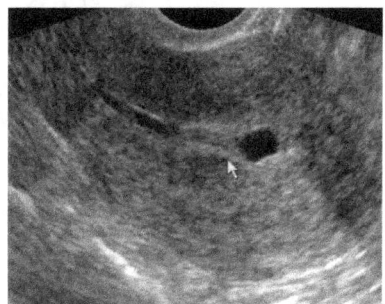

Submucous Fibroid   **Intrauterine Adhesions**

Saline Infusion Sonography (SIS)

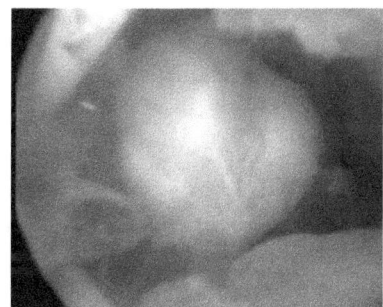
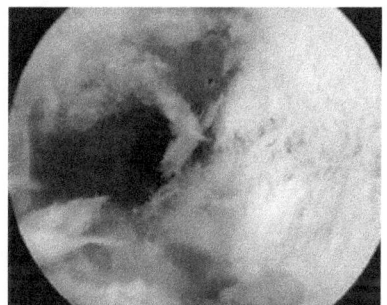

Submucous Fibroid   **Intrauterine Adhesions**

Hysteroscopy

TREATMENT

Treatment plans are based on the diagnosis, duration of infertility, and the woman's age.

Management of female factors may include medical treatment, surgical intervention, or assisted reproductive techniques.

Ovarian Factors

Treatment of ovarian factors may be medical (eg, pharmacotherapy) or surgical (eg, ovarian drilling).

Induction of Ovulation

Ovulation induction is the appropriate treatment for infertile patients who have dysfunction of the hypothalamic-pituitary-ovarian axis.

−Clomiphene Citrate (CC)

−Tamoxifen

−Aromatase Inhibitors

−Dopamine Agonists

−Human Menopausal Gonadotropins (hMG)

−Human Chorionic Gonadotropins (hCG)

−Gonadotropin Releasing Hormone (GnRH)

−Gonadotropin Releasing Hormone (GnRH) Antagonists

Treatment of Polycystic Ovarian Syndrome (PCOS)

Weight loss for obese women is important, not only for improving chances of ovulation, but also for reducing the risks during pregnancy.

CC is the first-line drug for treatment of anovulation.

Metformin is an insulin-sensitizing agent that has been used with off-label indication in the treatment of PCOS.

Gonadotropin therapy for ovulation induction in women with PCOS has been shown to be successful with pregnancy rates of approximately 22%.

Ovarian drilling involves drilling 3 to 10 holes per ovary at laparoscopy using electrocautery or laser.

Risks of the surgery include ovarian adhesions and ovarian failure if too many holes are drilled.

Treatment of Prolactinomas

Medical therapy involves the use of dopamine agonists to suppress prolactin secretion.

The most commonly used dopamine agonist is bromocriptine.

Cabergoline is a newer option and has fewer side effects.

Once the prolactin level is normalized, ovulation will be restored within a few months.

Macroadenomas can be treated medically, but surgery is often the preferred method for large masses.

Tubal Factors

Tubal reconstruction was the only hope for those patients before assisted reproductive therapy became available.

<u>Tubal Surgery</u>

Tubal obstruction and adhesions can be corrected through laparotomy, operative laparoscopy, and, in special circumstances, through operative hysteroscopy and tubal cannulation.

Lysis of adhesions should be meticulous, using hydrodissection and fine instruments.

Treatment of hydrosalpinx (distal tubal obstruction) with salpingostomy can be performed through microsurgery or operative laparoscopy.

If the fallopian tubes are beyond repair, bilateral salpingectomy with destruction of the cornual area is recommended in preparation for IVF.

<u>Assisted Reproduction Techniques (ART)</u>

ART used to treat infertility include the following:

– Intrauterine insemination (IUI).

– In vitro fertilization (IVF).

– Gamete intrafallopian transfer (GIFT).

– Zygote intrafallopian transfer (ZIFT).

– Intracytoplasmic sperm injection (ICSI).

Treatment of Endometriosis

Endometriosis treatment may be divided according to the severity of the disease and patient needs.

Four alternatives are currently available to treat endometriosis:

−Expectant therapy should be based on a complete workup with diagnosis of very early stages of the disease (minimal) in patients without clinical symptoms, ie, an incidental finding.

−Surgical treatment should be directed at destroying the disease using electrocoagulation, laser vaporization, endocoagulation, or excision.

−Medical treatment is directed toward suppressing estrogen production by the ovary with oral contraceptives, progestins, androgens (eg, danazol), or GnRH agonists (eg, Leuprolide acetate).

−Combined medical and surgical treatments are usually used for the treatment of severe endometriosis.

Uterine Factors

Surgical management of uterine factor infertility includes laparotomy, laparoscopy, or hysteroscopy.

Septate Uterus

Uterine anomalies can be corrected through operative hysteroscopy under general anesthesia or conscious sedation.

Furthermore, laparoscopy assists in the differential diagnosis between a septate and a bicornuate uterus.

Uterine Synechiae

Uterine synechiae are corrected using operative hysteroscopy; in many instances, more than one hysteroscopy is required.

Endometrial Polyps

Endometrial polyps are removed through operative hysteroscopy associated with a dilatation and curettage, if necessary.

Uterine Fibroids

Three modalities are used to treat myomas:

− Medical treatment is a temporary treatment, ideally used for patients who are close to menopause or who are risky surgical candidates.

− Surgical treatment of myomas includes conventional laparotomy, operative laparoscopy, and operative hysteroscopy.

− Uterine fibroid embolization consists of catheterization of the uterine artery and the injection of microbeads of polyvinyl alcohol to selectively occlude the circulation of the fibroid.

REFERENCES

– American Society for Reproductive Medicine. Use of clomiphene citrate in women. ASRM Committee Opinion. Fertil Steril. 2006; 86: S187-93.

– American Society for Reproductive Medicine. Use of exogenous gonadotropins in anovulatory women. ASRM Technical Bulletin. Fertil Steril. 2008; 90: S7-12.

– American Society for Reproductive Medicine. Gonadotropin preparations: past, present, and future perspectives. ASRM Educational Bulletin. Fertil Steril. 2008; 90: S13-20.

– Badawy A, Mosbah A, Tharwat A, et al. Extended letrozole therapy for ovulation induction in clomiphene-resistant women with polycystic ovary syndrome: a novel protocol. Fertil Steril. 2009; 92: 236-9.

– Barnhart K, Dunsmoor-Su R, Coutifaris C. Effect of endometriosis on in vitro fertilization. Fertil Steril. 2002: 77; 1148-55.

– Bedaiwy M, Mousa N, Esfandiari N, et al. Follicular phase dynamics with combined aromatase inhibitor and follicle stimulating hormone treatment. J Clin Endocrinol Metab. 2007; 92: 825-33.

– Berin I, Stein D, Keltz M. A comparison of gonadotropin-releasing hormone (GnRH) antagonist and GnRH agonist flare protocols for poor responders undergoing in vitro fertilization. Fertil Steril. 2010; 93: 360-3.

– Bhasin S, Mallidis C, Ma K. The genetic basis of infertility in men. Baillieres Best Pract Res Clin Endocrinol Metab. 2000; 14: 363-388.

– Brackett N, Lynne C, Aballa T, et al. Sperm motility from the vas deferens of spinal cord injured men is higher than from the ejaculate. J Urol. 2000; 164: 712-5.

– Broekmans F, Kwee J, Hendriks D, et al. A systematic review of tests predicting ovarian reserve and IVF outcome. Hum Reprod Update. 2006; 12: 685-718.

– Brugh V, Lipshultz L. Male factor infertility. Medical Clinics of North America. 2004; 88: 367-85.

– Buckingham K, Chamley L. A critical assessment of the role of antiphospholipid antibodies in infertility. J Reprod Immunol. 2009: 80; 132-45.

– Caburet S, Arboleda V, Llano E, et al. Mutant Cohesin in Premature Ovarian Failure. N Engl J Med. 2014; 370: 943-9.

– Carmignani L, Gadda F, Mancini M, et al. Detection of testicular ultrasonographic lesions in severe male infertility. J Urol. 2004; 172: 1045-7.

– Casper R, Mitwally M. Aromatase inhibitors for ovulation induction. J Clin Endocrinol Metab. 2006; 91: 760-71.

– Cavallini G. Male idiopathic oligoasthenoteratozoospermia. Asian Journal of Andrology. 2006; 8: 143-57.

– Centers for Disease Control and Prevention, American Society for Reproductive Medicine, Society for Assisted Reproductive Technology. 2006 Assisted Reproductive Technology Success Rates: National Summary and Fertility Clinic Reports, Atlanta: U.S. Department of Health and Human Services, Centers for Disease Control and Prevention; 2008.

– Chamley L, Clarke G. Antisperm antibodies and conception. Semin Immunopathol. 2007: 29; 169-84.

– Chung K. Gross Anatomy. 4th ed. Philadelphia: Lippincott Williams & Wilkins; 2000.

– Cline A, Kutteh W. Is there a role of autoimmunity in implantation failure after in-vitro fertilization? Curr Opin Obstet Gynecol. 2009: 21; 291-5.

– Daya S. Updated meta-analysis of recombinant follicle-stimulating hormone (FSH) versus urinary FSH for ovarian stimulation in assisted reproduction. Fertil Steril. 2002; 77: 711-4.

– Donckers J, Evers J, Land J. The long-term outcome of 946 consecutive couples visiting a fertility clinic in 2001-2003. Fertil Steril. 2011; 96: 160-4.

– Dovey S, Sneeringer R, Penzias A. Clomiphene citrate and intrauterine insemination: analysis of more than 4100 cycles. Fertil Steril. 2008; 90: 2281-6.

– Drake R, Vogl A, Mitchell A. Gray's Anatomy for Student's. 2nd ed. Philadelphia: Churchill Livingstone Elsevier; 2010.

– Eisenberg M, Betts P, Herder D, et al. Increased risk of cancer among azoospermic men. Fertil Steril. 2013; 100: 681-5.

– García-Ulloa A, Arrieta O. Tubal occlusion causing infertility due to an excessive inflammatory response in patients with predisposition for keloid formation. Med. Hypotheses 2005; 65: 908–14.

– Gillen-water J, Grayhack J, Howards S, et al, editors. Adult and pediatric urology. 4th ed. London: Lippincott. Williams & Wilkins; 2002.

– Gray H. Anatomy, Descriptive and Surgical. The Unabridged Gray's Anatomy. Philadelphia: Running Press; 1999.

– Hauser R, Yogev L, Paz G, et al. Comparison of efficacy of two techniques for testicular sperm retrieval in nonobstructive azoospermia. J Androl. 2006; 27: 28-33.

– Hirsh A. Male subfertility. BMJ. 2003; 327: 669-72.

– Huang H, Lv C, Zhao Y, et al. Mutant ZP1 in Familial Infertility. N Engl J Med. 2014; 370: 1220-6.

– Hwang K, Walters R, Lipshultz L. Contemporary concepts in the evaluation and management of male infertility. Nature Reviews Urology. 2011; 8: 86-94.

– Imani B, Eijkemans M, te Velde E, et al. A nomogram to predict the probability of live birth after clomiphene citrate induction of ovulation in normogonadotropic oligoamenorrheic infertility. Fertil Steril. 2002; 77: 91-7.

– Kallio S, Aittomäki K, Piltonen T, et al. Anti-Mullerian hormone as a predictor of follicular reserve in ovarian insufficiency: special emphasis on FSH-resistant ovaries. Hum Reprod. 2012; 27: 854-60.

– Katz V, Lentz G, Lobo R, et al. Comprehensive Gynecology. 5th ed. Philadelphia: Mosby Elsevier; 2007.

– Keel B. Within- and between-subject variation in semen parameters in infertile men and normal semen donors. Fertil Steril. 2006; 85: 128-34.

– Kim M, Kim N, Kim H, et al. Pregnancy following uterine artery embolization with polyvinyl alcohol particles for patients with uterine fibroid or adenomyosis. Cardiovasc Intervent Radiol. 2005; 28: 611-5.

– Koning A, Kuchenbecker W, Groen H, et al. Economic consequences of overweight and obesity in infertility: a framework for evaluating the costs and outcomes of fertility care. Hum Reprod Update. 2010; 16: 246-54.

– Legro R, Barnhart H, Schlaff W, et al. Cooperative Multicenter Reproductive Medicine Network. Clomiphene, metformin, or both for infertility in the polycystic ovary syndrome. N Engl J Med. 2007; 356: 551-66.

– Lombardo F, Sansone A, Romanelli F, et al. The role of antioxidant therapy in the treatment of male infertility: An overview. Asian Journal of Andrology. 2011; 13: 690-7.

– Lord J, Flight I, Norman R. Metformin in polycystic ovary syndrome: systematic review and meta-analysis. BMJ. 2003; 327: 951-3.

– Loukas M, Colburn G, Abrahams P, et al. Gray's Anatomy Review. Philadelphia: Churchill Livingstone Elsevier; 2010.

– Macklon D, Fauser C. Medical approaches to ovarian stimulation for infertility. In: Jerome F. Strauss I, Robert L. Barbieri M, eds. Yen & Jaffe's Reproductive Endocrinology, 6th Edition Vol. 28. Philadelphia: Saunders, 2009: 698-708.

– Magos A. Hysteroscopic treatment of Asherman's syndrome. Reprod Biomed Online. 2002; 4: S46-51.

– Male Infertility Best Practice Policy Committee of the American Urological Association; Practice Committee of the ASRM. Report on optimal evaluation of the infertile male. Fertil Steril. 2006; 86: S202-9.

– Mills J, Meacham R. Nonsurgical Treatment of male infertility. In Lipshultz L, Howards S, and Niederberger C (eds). Infertility in the Male, 4th ed. Cambridge: Cambridge University Press; 2009.

– Neill J. Knobil and Neill's Physiology of Reproduction. 3rd ed. St. Louis, MO: Elsevier; 2006.

– Ovalle W, Nahirney P. Netter's Eseential Histology. Philadelphia: Sauders Elsevier; 2007.

– Palomba S, Orio F, Falbo A, et al. Clomiphene citrate versus metformin as first-line approach for the treatment of anovulation in infertile patients with polycystic ovary syndrome. J Clin Endocrinol Metab. 2007; 92: 3498-503.

– Practice Committee of the American Society for Reproductive Medicine. Endometriosis and Infertility. Fertil Steril. 2006; 86: S156-60.

– Practice Committee of the American Society for Reproductive Medicine. Report on management of obstructive azoospermia. Fertil Steril. 2006; 86: S259-63.

– Practice Committee of the American Society for Reproductive Medicine. Optimal evaluation of the infertile female. Fertil Steril. 2006; 86: S264-7.

– Practice Committee of American Society for Reproductive Medicine in collaboration with Society for Reproductive Endocrinology and Infertility. Optimizing natural fertility. Fertil Steril. 2008; 90: S1-6.

– Practice Committee of the American Society for Reproductive Medicine. Current Evaluation of amenorrhea. Fertil Steril. 2008; 90: S219-25.

– Reindollar R, Regan M, Neumann P, et al. A randomized clinical trial to evaluate optimal treatment for unexplained infertility: the fast track and standard treatment (FASTT) trial. Fertil Steril. 2010; 94: 888-99.

– Rosendahl M, Andersen C, La Cour Freiesleben N, et al. Dynamics and mechanisms of chemotherapy-induced ovarian follicular depletion in women of fertile age. Fertil Steril. 2010; 94: 156-66.

– Rotterdam ESHRE/ASRM-Sponsored PCOS Consensus Workshop Group. Revised 2003 consensus on diagnostic criteria and long-term health risks related to polycystic ovary syndrome. Fertil Steril. 2004; 81: 19-25.

– Sadler T. Langman's Medical Embryology. 11th ed. Baltimore, Maryland: Lippincott Williams & Wilkins; 2010.

– Speroff L, Fritz M, eds. Clinical Gynecologic Endocrinology and Infertility, 7th edition. Philadelphia: Lippincot, Williams & Wilkins, 2005.

– Standring S. Gray's Anatomy. 40th ed. Edinburgh: Elsevier Churchill Livingstone; 2008.

– Sun W, Stegmann B, Henne M, et al. A new approach to ovarian reserve testing. Fertil Steril. 2008; 90: 2196-202.

– Ten Broek R, Kok-Krant N, Bakkum E, et al. Different surgical techniques to reduce post-operative adhesion formation: A systematic review and meta-analysis. Hum Reprod Update. 2012; 19: 12-25.

– The Evian Annual Reproduction (EVAR) Workshop Group 2010; Fauser BCJM, Diedrich K, Bouchard P, et al. Contemporary genetic technologies and female reproduction. Hum Reprod Update. 2011; 17: 829-47.

– Thessaloniki ESHRE/ASRM – Sponsored PCOS Consensus Workshop Group. Consensus on infertility treatment related to polycystic ovary syndrome. Human Reprod. 2008; 23: 462-77.

– Traber M, Stevens J. Vitamins C and E: Beneficial effects from a mechanistic perspective. Free Radical Biology and Medicine. 2011; 51: 1000-13.

– Tur-Kaspa I, Gal M, Hartman M, et al. A prospective evaluation of uterine abnormalities by saline infusion sonohysterography in 1,009 women with infertility or abnormal uterine bleeding. Fertil Steril. 2006; 86: 1731-5.

– Vicdan A, Vicdan K, Günalp S, et al. Genetic aspects of human male infertility: the frequency of chromosomal abnormalities and Y chromosome microdeletions in severe male factor infertility. Eur J Obstet Gynecol Reprod Biol. 2004; 117: 49-54.

– Wang J, Zhang W, Jiang H, et al. Mutations inHFM1in Recessive Primary Ovarian Insufficiency. N Engl J Med. 2014; 370: 972-4.

– Wein A. Campbell-Walsh Urology. 9th ed. Philadelphia: Saunders Elsevier; 2007.

– Whitten S, Nangia A, Kolettis P. Select patients with hypogonadotropic hypogonadism may respond to treatment with clomiphene citrate. Fertil Steril. 2006; 86: 1664-8.

– World Health Organization (WHO). Laboratory Manual for the Examination and Processing of Human Semen. 5th Edition. Geneva, Switzerland: World Health Organization (WHO); 2010.

www.ingramcontent.com/pod-product-compliance
Lightning Source LLC
Chambersburg PA
CBHW071229220526
45468CB00002B/775